MW01115550

"To Dr. Louis Jordan, a brilliant surgeon, pioneer and visionary.
The starting point he provided led to the book you have in your hands.
My patients have all benefited from his foresight and insight.
His medical practice was exemplary.
Men of his caliber will be sorely missed in times to come."

Medical Disclaimer:

Address Inquiries to:
Stiles Rehab, LLC
2175 Bullis Rd
Elma, NY 14059

Contents

Prologue

My Story

Living in Virginia Beach and spending my weekends at the beach playing volleyball from sun up to almost sundown: I was in the midst of changing jobs. I can't even recall what precipitated the change but I found myself caring for the patients of Dr. Louis Jordan, an orthopedic surgeon at the forefront of perfecting a rapidly expanding surgery at the time, the total knee replacement. It was the early 90's. To be honest, when I heard about his protocol for the new knees I was a bit skeptical, thinking it would be too hard on the patients. Well I was about to be schooled, as they say. I learned a bunch in that time that I have now expanded upon, but there was no one I encountered who was as forward thinking and hands down correct about the total knee rehabilitation as Dr. Jordan.

Now as I look back on an almost 20 year career in 5 different states and hundreds of total knee patients later, I realize that plenty of the nuggets and tips that I know and use daily are still not regularly practiced in the field today. My learning lab, which has been the patient one-on-one in the home, has afforded me a unique opportunity to ruthlessly cut out what doesn't work and retain the minimal essential tools that will get the job done in the fastest way possible. At the core, I am a realist. People only have so much time and energy that can be devoted to rehab and beyond that they have lives that need to be lived.

Why am I bothering to mention all that? Really just to give you some background on what makes me tick and why you might listen to what I have to say. I avoid "medicalese speak" like the plague. Plain English is what you will find here and hopefully you will feel empowered to oversee your own progress, enlightened and confident that you know the way and demystified of many of the sacred cows of the medical system.

One more note about what this book is and is not. It's not a treatise on osteoarthritis, or the broad scope of knee surgeries. It is not a detailed description of the different surgical techniques and implants used in the total knee category, nor a compendium of all possible exercises that you could possibly do following your surgery. It is a defined system utilizing select principles that will get you through the total knee rehab with the least possible pain, effort and time commitment - and who doesn't want that?

"May your journey be fulfilling as you help others along the way."

Michelle PT

Origins of a Tool

My Father had been ill and I relocated back up to the western New York area to be closer to home. Now I was back in the field working and everyone was coming out of the hospitals with-of all things-rolling walkers. I was working almost exclusively on total knee patients on a daily basis and was annoyed that I had lost my very best weapon. When I was in Virginia, as per MD orders, we had been instructed to turn the standard walker (no wheels) sideways, have the patient place his or her foot on the cross bar and then using arms only, leverage the walker back toward the knee. Yes, it was cumbersome; at times the walker did not fit within confined spaces easily, the cross bars were frequently higher than patients would have liked and, yes, you are exactly right in thinking that it was not particularly easy to get buy in from many of the patients. Sure they questioned our sanity, our IQ's, our motivation and certainly last but not least our compassion. After all, this is not how their neighbor's rehab had gone. Everyone in his right mind in the early 90's knew you needed time to rest before your really tested the limits of a surgical knee.

Where was Dr. Jordan when you needed him? My patients were driving me nuts. The change in walker preference was dictated by a change in surgical procedure from bone ingrowth system which the MD's felt demanded protected weight-bearing to a preference for cemented systems where the patient could more quickly enjoy weight-bearing as tolerated. Standard walkers were almost never issued and I was without my best tool.

By nature I tend to be a bit high strung. I like success and progress toward goals. Time and again, despite my best efforts, I would revisit a patient only to inform him that he had declined or made no progress since my last visit. Being driven crazy with stagnant results, I would redouble my efforts in teaching the exercises and principles. Quite honestly, however, we had meager resources in the home with which to promote knee range.

We were no longer using continuous passive motion (CPM) machines in Virginia and New York. As soon as a few studies had come out stating that the progress gained with a CPM machine was short lived compared to those who had not used it-well that was all the insurance companies needed to hear. Now that wasn't all bad, because some people really got into bad habits using the CPM and thinking that it was up to the machine to "fix' them. You know that is not going to go well.

So then what do you have? The classic sitting chair single leg slide, where a patient "scrubs the floor," thereby promoting range of motion of the surgical knee. Sometimes a towel is placed under the foot for less friction and better glide. Also we have the exercise where a patient lies on his back and tries to pull the heel up toward the body by itself at first, and then assisted by some other means like a towel, sheet, belt or leg strap. Oh boy, doesn't that sound like fun.

Gentle rocking in a rocking chair or swinging the leg on the back of a pickup truck or tall table are two other methods. Note to self: must buy a pickup truck next time I trade my car in to cheerfully help my patients. Maybe I can get a tax break.

It must seem like a pretty obvious conclusion: the humble home is not the best place for rehab. Surely when a patient gets to all the high tech sparkling rehab gadgets he thinks that things will go much better. Stationary bikes, Nu-step machines, mini-bikes, therapy balls, weight machines and such, sounds like rehab nirvana. All the tools, all the very best rehab the 21st century can afford. Oh, but wait... there's a catch. There is a fly in that ointment; a very serious flaw.

As a home care therapist without access to the bells and whistles of outpatient rehab, was I likely to be annoyed day in and day out by inconsistent progress? Two things bothered me. The patients down in Virginia had been very successful. I seriously wondered if I would have to look for different work, things had gotten so easy. The other thought that made me uneasy was the genuine look in people's eyes when they told me, "But I did my exercises, really." After a number of years working in rehab it's fairly easy to detect, well, let's not call them "liars," but those patients who aren't quite adequately reflecting their true home exercise program effort.

Then one day I had an idea that seemed sacrilegious at the time. I had an old walker in my shed and decided to take the hack saw to it, cutting the side panel off. I had never destroyed a walker before! Having done that, I was now looking at a jagged section of metal sticking out, well that's not going to work, I thought. I went and got the metal file and set to work. When I had done all I could do, I knew it still would not pass a safety test. So of course I did what all single women do when they can't do any better. I grabbed a roll of duct tape and slapped it around that tubing to the tune of .5 inch thickness and bam! It was done. It did not look anything like a glittering, high tech, professional tool, in fact, it looked quite ugly, but I knew it would work and that is all that mattered.

Now about this same time, I had added a technique to the classic "single leg chair slides" that I felt improved its effectiveness. First of all it is necessary to have a floor surface on which a patient's foot will glide: wood, tile, or linoleum is pretty much it, and in many cases these surfaces are in a kitchen or hallway. I wanted a method that would give my patents an objective measuring tool with which they could monitor their progress.

If you put masking tape down on the floor, put the chair up to the wall and left it there, the whole thing was pretty much standardized and thereby a useful technique for giving range of motion feedback. What I had done was exchange degrees measured by a goniometer that only a PT could read, for marks on the floor (inches in other words) that anyone could read.

Sounds great, doesn't it? God bless the spouses that had to put up with me. In many cases the floor surface held a lot of friction. In an effort to help some struggling patients I would put powder down on the floor to create a friction-free surface. Bingo, worked like a charm, but weary caregivers were not particularly enthralled with the idea. Not that it bothered me too much; I was seeing consistent progress. Yippee! They were also equally unenthusiastic about the idea of putting masking tape down on a good wood floor. I couldn't blame them. A compromise was reached, and in the end, I used a yardstick as a measuring tool laid down on the floor instead of tape.

Everything's hunky-dory right? No, because now caregivers complained that they don't want a chair to stay permanently in the kitchen or hallway area. For crying out loud, did they make my job hard! Here I am and all I'm trying to do is help. Then one day it happened: a man that I would like to nominate as caregiver of the decade if there were such a thing, got so fed up with my nonsense that he went in the garage tore down a simple corrugated box so that it was about the length of a yardstick, took some old roofing flashing (silver metal that is a nice friction free surface) cut it up and duct taped it to the cardboard. Viola! No more powder on the floor, no more tape on the floor, a portable sliding tool that can be picked up easily and gotten out of the way if need be.

I sat in stunned silence. It was the answer I had been looking for. In another week or two I had made my first template out of a sturdy wooden bottom, the metal flashing edges now being safely tucked away under wooden 1/4 rounds at the ends and two yardsticks that went up and down the length.

I used to lovingly call my hacked up side of a walker "the Rack". Of course it didn't really look like a 16th century torture device, but it was fun to tease. Patients' first impressions were very skeptical at first and I had to do my best teacher-trainer, selling tactics to get them to understand the incredible value and the secret to success that they now held in their hands.

These days, I have a more professional looking model. It still takes time for people to warm up to it, but in the end, most people wish to continue using it longer than their home care frequency allows. Occasionally, if someone really wanted if someone wanted to keep the hacked up side of the walker tool then I would barter. If they had or could find an old walker for me, we could trade. My patients would continue to use the tool to their benefit and I would get two new ones, once the demolition of the old walker took place.

So there you have the beginnings of the Fast Track Total Knee System. In it's infancy, the system was still mostly two tools, but as time went by, I began to identify the powerful principles that I believe fuel its success. It soon became very clear how relatively easy it was to get full range of motion back post surgically in 2-3 weeks if you followed the right template.

But before we get into the meat and taters, so to speak, follow me if you will on a short detour about the tale of two masters.

A Tale of Two Masters

What I have found as I have travelled around doing physical therapy in 5 different states is that the approach to total knee rehab is "essentially the same" but wildly different in results and outcomes. I see people who come out of the hospital with 65 degrees range of motion and 93 degrees range of motion. How can this be? Look the phrase "total knee rehab" up on the Internet and most every page will say the same thing. How is it that the results are so different and that the subjective experience varies so much? Everyone has heard stories of Aunt Millie who no longer walks right or never got off the walker again after her surgery, and others who are back to work and golf in short order.

There are, in my opinion, six hallmarks of an exceptional rehab enterprise and seven silver bullets of rehab success that I will explain further on in the book. When these are aligned, the total knee rehab experience is relatively painless and proceeds quickly through defined benchmarks. It is however a rather narrowly defined path through pitfalls, scrub brush and sharp overhangs that you should avoid. If a patient strays from the path, things can get ugly fast and then this surgical procedure becomes a lengthy ordeal that he cannot conceive of ever attempting again. Short note here: In the first three days after surgery, 95% of my patients are questioning their decision to have gone ahead with the surgery. If I don't help them find the path out of pain and endless swelling fast, negative thoughts and frustrations set in and discourage the patient.

Let me give you a comparative example, using the game of golf. There are certain things you must master to be a good golfer: the drive, short game, putting, etc. It would be relatively easy to find the content related to how to drive the ball properly, how to hit using a 7 iron, or how to hold the putter and analyze the green. It is another thing entirely to have at your disposal, the frequency, order of focus, essential feedback and the structured advance of training that the pros use. As they say, the devil is in the details, and the details I've found are critical. What I aim to give you here is the wisdom that only a seasoned professional can give. Fortunately, getting your knee flexion and strength back is not nearly as hard as mastering the game of golf.

By a lucky twist of fate, I've had the chance in my career to work one on one with hundreds of patients struggling to get their knee back in shape after a total knee replacement. Had I not been in home care, and had I not had the good fortune of working rather directly with a few orthopedic MDs who were demanding and paternalistic regarding their rehab results, I probably would not be able to give you the knowledge that I do today.

For the most part today in rehab settings, whether it is sub acute or outpatient, therapists are managing essentially capped by the government, the only way to make more money is to see more patients. I frequently tell people that in healthcare we serve two masters, you the patient and the payee.

The payee drives the paperwork and the regulations surrounding the all-important topic of getting paid or reimbursed. This is the second evil master at work simply by virtue of us having a third party payer system. Ostensively, your welfare is of paramount importance to them. In reality, we get paid when we deliver the paperwork the way they want it in a timely manner. We do not get paid for delivering great care. The burdens of the payee requirements unfortunately drive the whole system. With the advent of computers, the corporate takeover of medicine and government interference, high quality direct care is becoming something of a novelty. You know I am telling you the truth because you have experienced it.

So my point in discussing this is not a rant on healthcare, but that you should know that now is the time to take control of your own health outcomes. Be responsible for yourself and less trusting of the people assigned to take care of you. Many of them are wonderful, many of them are overworked and many are simply assigned duties that are becoming less and less essential for you the patient. If your healthcare professional stinks or the facility is lousy, it's probably because they have decided that their job is easier if they concentrate on serving the payee instead of you. To attempt to serve both well is difficult and at times exhausting. There is inherent conflict and I myself have been worn out by it. I remember some biblical verse regarding serving two masters and, as I recall, it didn't work out well in the end.

Interestingly the American Physical Therapy Association (APTA) did an in-depth study of the state of the art of total knee rehab in 2010. Hughes (2010) made a stunning admission in the monograph.

The outcomes of excellent ROM and the ability to ambulate and self-progress with home exercise are universal; the most efficient and cost effective way to achieve these goals remains elusive. (p. 29)

The first total knee was performed in 1950's but the modern total knee with which we are familiar was coming into its own back in the early 1990's. Twenty years of rehab later, the best total knee rehab is elusive. Hughes (2010) also stated that "identifying appropriate levels of rapid progressions to minimize postoperative impairments and complications will undoubtedly characterize the 2010 decade in TKA rehabilitation."(p. 29)

Rehabilitation guidelines and benchmarks for total knee replacement recovery were created out of a study conducted in 2005 at the University of Delaware. The chart below summarizes how the Fast Track system compares with the industry standards on the parameter of range of motion.

Rehabilitation guidelines and benchmarks for total knee replacement recovery were created out of a study conducted in 2005 at the University of Delaware.

The chart below summarizes how the Fast Track System compares with the industry standards on the parameter of Range of motion

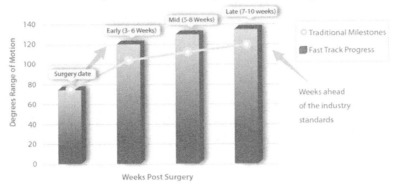

So my take on it is this: if the present state of rehab generates inconsistent results, and the APTA even admits to not knowing how to do this well, then it behooves you to at least listen to the thoughts and comments contained in this book related to my considerable experience in the field of total knee replacement recovery. You won't be sorry.

The Heart of the Matter

The Six Hallmarks of a Successful Total Knee Rehab
Enterprise

The six hallmarks of a successful total knee rehab enterprise
include pre-surgical education, excellent hospital push, a coordinated
rehab system, consistent early narcotic pain use, structured incremental
recovery, live time feedback and easily accessible leverage. I will briefly
discuss each of them here.

PRE-SURGICAL EDUCATION

Enhancing brain function is not one of the intended effects or unintended
side effects of narcotic pain med use. Because of this fact, it is highly
beneficial to be engaged in pre-surgical education of the rehab process.
Knowing what you will be asked to do, how to do those things and
what to have in advance in the home setting is really, really valuable.
Caregivers and others that will be assisting you, like spouse or children,
can get the training as well. Reading this short book will go a long way
to putting everyone on the same page. It is not optimal if the first time
you hear about a flex bar and what it can do for you is after your surgery
with your head foggy from narcotic substances.

EXCELLENT HOSPITAL PUSH

A strong hospital thrust can scale down your rehab time by almost a full
week. This is critically important for all those 50-60 year old folks who
need to get back to work in 4 to 6 weeks or anyone else who just values
their time in life. What do I mean by a thrust? I mean specifically:
advancing your knee bend. Sad to say that in many places the therapist
just gets you up walking, and makes sure you can get in and out of bed
and up and down stairs. You are on your own to advance your continuous
passive motion machine (hereafter CPM) to increase your range of
motion or for that matter do any other exercises to advance your range of
motion.

19

Without support and education most people will easily succumb to the idea that they should be very obliging to the knee early. Why? Because it is swollen, looks terrible and the incision might split open and boy they would be in a terrible mess then. This is a commonplace and reasonable reaction. However, the real deal is that in reality you will never be more medicated than at this stage. Use it to your utmost advantage by pushing that knee range as high as you can get it. Dominate early and make your future rehab rock.

A COORDINATED REHAB SYSTEM

This is so critical. There are situations where a patient will have a hospital therapist for 1-3 days, then a home therapist for 2 weeks and then another therapist in the outpatient setting.

If they are all saying the same things this is great. Everyone on the same page and the patient is not confused or discouraged. When this is not the case I really feel sorry for the patient who is trying to navigate conflicting advice. Who should they believe and trust most in a very critical time for them?

CONSISTENT EARLY NARCOTIC PAIN USE

Now I absolutely know that this is the one piece of advice that patients resist the most. So I will give you my caveat in advance. I am about the most adamant person you will find against taking medication for anything, my default setting is to try any other method possible to alleviate symptoms or fix conditions. Just ask my mother. She will tell you how I am constantly getting her to rethink a medication solution compared with other alternatives. Why would I "push" medicine?

Ironically, taking your pain medicine as prescribed initially is the fastest way to get off them. Let me say that again because it bears repeating. If you follow the advice as given you can be off pain medicine in 2-3 weeks and be able to switch to an over the counter medicine. You will take less overall in the long run than if you take them sparingly. I guarantee you, taking them niggardly in the beginning will not only wreck your progress in rehab, but will result in you taking more pain medicine because you will be on them for much longer.

Recently, I had to undergo an appendectomy and they placed me on narcotic pain medicine after the surgery. Despite being in significant pain prior to the surgery I had elected not to take pain medicine. I had an inkling I might be in the category of people who do not tolerate them well (i.e. get sick when sitting up) because of my genetics. It turns out I was right. This has helped to create a new found dose of empathy for my patients who are in a similar situation.

Anecdotally, I would say that about 3-5% of my patients are in this predicament following a total knee surgery. If you are nauseous when taking your pain medicine, it will be hard for you to complete the exercises. How will you make progress? I have found that most people in this category can tolerate the medicine better if they can cut them in half and take small quantities frequently throughout the day. In addition there are other anti-nausea pills that can help as well.

STRUCTURED INCREMENTAL RECOVERY

What do I mean by this strange phrase? There are certain things you should focus on first then second then third. Mess up this order and you are going to start wandering into the brush, wondering when in the heck this is going to get better. This is a perversely common error. Focus! Order! Structure! First work on this and then work on the next object of focus. I will explain exactly what I mean in a future section. Also the recovery needs to be incremental. I have found there is a certain speed at which we can progress. If you transgress and get too greedy, your body will punish you. Delay will result and you are back at square one before you got greedy.

THE SEVEN SILVER BULLETS OF SUCCESS

The seven silver bullets of success are the principles I use to advance the rehab process in a very structured, methodical and systematic way. By virtue of this being a system, it is highly repeatable. When my patients return for a second total knee replacement, they are well equipped to apply this system to the new rehab situation. All I do is remind and reinforce. They do not look to me to "fix" them. Patients come into the next surgery knowing they have control and knowing they will be successful.

21

It's like putting the patient on autopilot. They understand how to do it themselves using the right tools and applying the principles. These principles are laid out for you in the next chapter.

The Seven Silver Bullets Of Success

The seven silver bullets of success are the principles that drive this system. It's the 'why', 'how' and "when" behind the 'what'. Seemingly everyone has the same exercises to start with, why the disparity of outcomes? It's because the exercises are just one/seventh of what you need to know. It is just one silver bullet. Each bullet added to the next causes an accelerator factor. If you do one of these only, there would not be a noticeable difference. Put them all together and the change is striking.

I had a therapist cover a total knee patient of mine who remarked in his notes that the patient's progress was exceptional. Her story is as follows: She came home from the hospital with 83 degrees range of motion post surgically and 15 days later she had 125. She was discharged to outpatient at her 2-week follow-up visit. She followed the script exactly and the end result was 2.6 degrees of progress a day. This is the usual result seen with this system, 2-3 degrees range of motion progress a day. There is no other system that I am aware, where progress with range of motion is consistently achieved. So let's get started.

FOCUS

The primary focus following a total knee surgery should be range of motion recovery. This seems highly unnatural and counterintuitive secondary to the swelling. Most people will be reluctant to bend the knee because it feels weird and they believe that they are going to hurt the knee. They also think that things will get better when the swelling goes down. In fact the repetitive motion of the knee actually helps to drive the swelling out of the leg incrementally at first and finally permanently. Waiting for the swelling to go down by itself would take far too long and delay your entire rehab progress.

This principle is so important that I structure 80% of the initial exercises around range of motion development. Human beings will tend to avoid the hard things. I narrow everything down until they get this part and understand how to make progress. At any time, the 20% other exercises can be omitted and flexion/extension sessions only assigned.

Walking without the walker should NOT be your focus, nor is it some kind of critical victory over the surgery. Walking again will NOT be your problem. In the early stages it will aggravate your swelling and delay the desired progress of range in your knee. You should be allowing your knee to have protected weight bearing, meaning you put some weight through your arms onto the walker for at least the first two weeks.

Putting your full body weight on a surgical knee is too much force for the new knee. All the structures are tender and will swell. On the other hand, bending does not involve gravity-like forces and is therapeutic. Staying on the walker, and using ice are the only ways I want you to pamper your knee. Don't pamper it in regard to the range.

Once you have the full range, or at least 120 degrees of flexion, you can ramp up the strength development. Remember, I am working on strength right from the beginning (these are the 20% exercises I mentioned earlier), but don't focus on it until after the range is well along and will readily abandon if the range progression is not adequate. First, you start on basic strength. Basic strength is just getting the limb to move through the full range followed by the full range against gravity. When a patient can do an anti-gravity exercise 20- 25 repetitions 4x a day, he is ready to use a lightweight (1-1.5 lb.) for that particular exercise, not necessarily the whole routine. The weights can be done on alternate sets in the beginning to increase tolerance to them.

A home ankle weight set is really essential. They can be purchased for $10-$20 and will keep you progressing at your maximal rate. If you don't get a weight set you will be wasting time with active range of motion exercises that will not be helping you get any stronger. Why do work that is a waste of time? When you have moved on to the outpatient setting where three times a week is the typical frequency, you will still have a weight set at home so you can continue to build strength on the "off " therapy days. This is the fastest way to success. Doing nothing on the off days is sure to extend your rehab time.

Once you have a foundation of basic strength you can move onto more body weight activities. These are usually in the standing position and include things like a mini lunge, chair squats, step ups, step downs and lateral steps. Remembering what was said earlier about weight bearing, you can now see why these cannot be started too early, as they will promote too much swelling. Here then is the order: Range of motion, basic strength, functional strength and walking. The graph shows approximate percentage of focus for the various stages of recovery during a post-surgical time period.

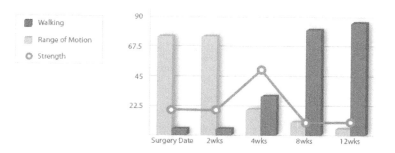

In the early stage (0- 2 or 3 weeks), range of motion is the primary focus. In the middle stage (3- 7 weeks), strength building is the primary focus. And in the final stage, walking and functional activities would be the main concern.

FREQUENCY

The name of the tool I will introduce to you later is "The FLEX bar" for Frequent Leveraged Exercise. Frequency is what will allow you to stay ahead of the swelling and probably is the most unrecognized critical element of success in the world of rehab today. Your assignment, if you choose to fast track your recovery, is to do your exercises four times a day. You will swell at night. Typically patients say they feel the worst in the morning. Your first session will be to drive out the overnight swelling, and in the morning you may only get back to baseline (what you achieved in your final session the night before). That is ok. In your next session you should feel better and be able to advance. Do the same with the third session. The fourth session is tougher. People are tired but if you can at least maintain the range you gained during the day, or advance a little, you will have been successful.

Now at this point you may feel that I have tricked you. I promised to accelerate your rehab with the least amount of effort and now I am assigning you a butt-kicking program frequency of four times a day. But wait, this frequency is what allows you to progress two to three degrees range of motion a day. By compressing your effort you will be highly successful and be "done" with your range work in 2-3 weeks. Being unable to bend your knee fully is what makes you feel "not over" your surgery. Kicking the range problem out of your way early makes a huge difference in your mental attitude and feeling of mastery over the situation, in addition to being the critical factor in allowing you to get off the narcotic pain medicine early.

If you follow the template you can gain success over the hard part, the thing that can linger on for 3- 6 months and make you wish you never had the knee surgery in the first place.

If you only do the exercises twice during the day, here's what will happen: First session, you drive the fluid out from the night time and then in your afternoon session some 6-8 hours later after accumulating essentially another nighttime of swelling, you will be doing well just to get that new swelling back out. You are on the treadmill of what I call "battling back to baseline," unable to generate any new range progress daily. This is what drives people crazy about this surgery and the associated recovery. They feel like losers. They do everything we say twice a day and it does not feel like they are getting ahead. In fact, by our exercise prescription we have doomed the patient to this frustration and madness.

Increasing the frequency allows you to "maintain the gain." After you manage to push some fluid out, you go back in another 1-3 hours and resume the same strategy, and you will begin to make incremental progress. This progress is 2-3 degrees per day of consistent advancement.

Being by nature a competitive person, at first this seemed discouraging. But in reality, it is the fastest a body can presently be pushed without creating a backlash of increased pain. What I have found is that the effort to accelerate this process by pushing the range to 4-6 degrees a day, will cause the patient to report a severe increase in pain that will prevent him from doing any of his exercises the next day. This results in a yo-yo effect; push hard one day and doing nothing the next. It is much more effective and more comfortable to the patient, to stay within the 2-3 degree range per day and be able to stay extremely consistent.

In my early days, I would help patients bend their knee (called active assisted motion, ((most people call it torture) and try to push to the limits of that days stretching. This is a precarious process secondary to the psychological dynamics that take place between two people and a potentially painful activity.

The patient does not want to appear wimpy or not "all in" and this can lead the therapist to think that they are tolerating it well but in time they are really hurting because they overdid it. At the other end of the spectrum is the patient who really isn't motivated and grimaces practically every time you touch his leg.

Of course each person has his own perception of what pain is and how much he is experiencing. I will talk later on in the book about how I solved this. Just realize that the therapist does not have a super human 6th sense for what level of assistance is just right and I almost never assist a patient in this manner any more.

FEEDBACK

This principle has been tested and proven in a multitude of disciplines and needs no endorsement from me. It does however need to be applied adequately to the challenge of rehabbing after a total knee. Now when I say feedback. I mean a measurable outcome that gives the patient an idea of whether his or her efforts are doing the trick or making progress toward a given goal. I do not mean to include verbal encouragement that tells a patient "Doing well. Keep it up."

Presently feedback is intermittent in the form of a therapist using a devise called a goniometer to measure your knee angle. This might occur daily in the home for a short time but then will occur only every few days when the patient has a PT session. In other words, the average patient is in the dark in determining whether each session is effective or not. They might have some generally vague sense that they are doing better one day from the next as noted by the stiffness in their knee, but no hard, fast evidence.

This is why I developed the tool called the Track. People get encouraged when they use this because they can actually see the progress toward their end goals and that will usually reenergize them to keep going. They also come to trust what I am telling them because inevitably if they follow the instructions their range keeps improving by 2-3 degrees per day. It is also invaluable in driving home my point about losing range and sliding back when the frequency dips. A patient might be doing well and think that they can cut corners and achieve the same progress, but the track does not

27

lie. When their frequency goes down they have to work all that much harder at the next session to get back to their baseline and they will realize that this is ultimately self-defeating. There are ways to mark measurable progress with almost every stretching exercise that I prescribe but usually all you have to do is measure one or two only and that is enough.

PROTECTION

Protection is a major goal of mine throughout the rehab process. I want my patients to feel confident so that 1. They are not going to hurt themselves and 2. I am not going to hurt them. So I teach them the incremental system of 1/2 inch more advance when they are using the Track. If someone is stuck at a certain knee range with their active pulls into flexion, I will always be able to ask them to move 1/2 inch further back and to hold that position for a count of 10-15 seconds. They may be a bit uncomfortable but will not experience sharp pain. I generally ask them to do 2 more holds of the same length and then go back to an active pull. This will usually propel them through the "stuck" zone and on into new range.

I do the same thing with the FLEX bar. I ask the patient to incrementally position the FLEX bar closer to them by about .5 inch. Then they work on loosening the bar up at this new level. I tell my patients that as long as they advance like this they will never "Ow" themselves with an exercise that I prescribe. If they receive a shockwave of pain, it is a signal that they have gone too far for any one particular session or gotten too aggressive with their progress.
Once a patient experiences an "Ow" or sharp pain that they recoil from, it creates a problem of trust. If the exercises I told them to do causes it, people will back off the exercises. If by assisting a knee bend I precipitate the "Ow", they will subconsciously tighten up when we attempt this in the future and no amount of coaching will correct it.

I categorically do not want my patients to experience sharp pain; it delays the rehab process, makes them worry about their knee being "hurt" and in general causes distrust of the whole rehab experience and personnel. On the other hand, I want to progress as fast as possible so that they can get beyond their rehab and get on with life. The system I have developed gives patients parameters and guidelines that assist them to get maximal stretching on the leg without the negative consequences of getting too aggressive and overdoing it, thereby causing pain.

LEVERAGE

There are two definitions of leverage that this system is utilizing. One is the mechanical advantage gained by being in a position to use a lever. The FLEX bar is a lever. The patient is able to use his arms through the mechanical advantage of the FLEX Bar to stretch the knee back. This tool allows the patient to sit upright in a comfortable position and easily leverage the knee back in a very controlled fashion. Patients are surprised at the power they have and are at first rather nervous, but after training and coaching they realize that they are in control and will be systematically, incrementally driving the fluid out of their knee.

There are plenty of ways that therapists have been using leverage but none so easy, accessible, and portable as this method, not to mention effective. The typical exercise that is given the patient is for him to lie on his back and try to bring his heel toward his upper body in the manner of a heel slide. A strap or long sheet can be used as the leverage to assist the pull up toward the body. This exercise drives me nuts. It is a terrible biomechanical position, there is no way to measure improvement and the leverage system is awkward at best. For years this is the best we can come up with?

A therapist could instruct the patient to use the other "good" leg to leverage the surgical leg back and this is somewhat effective but not if the other leg is in poor condition. Also it should be noted that a leg does not have as fine a motor control as the upper extremities and therefore it is more likely that the patient will overshoot (causing pain) while assisting with the leg.

A patient can use stairs as a type of leverage system. Leaning your body over the knee with your foot on a stair step leverages the body weight to force the knee bend. I however, would rate this exercise to have a rather high degree of difficulty. Technically it is harder to master and easier to fudge (look like you are achieving something by substituting movement from somewhere else, like the hip), not to mention the problems with putting some older adults on one leg secondary to balance issues and the practical problems with finding a suitable staircase upon which to do the exercises safely.

Tools that can be found in an outpatient clinic can only be used several times a week, so clearly following the discussion of frequency this is unsuitable. I would like to mention another leverage technique to improve range of motion, and that is using a stationary bike. The leverage used in this method is both powerful and poorly controlled, which is why I do not recommend using this at all. When you have the other leg generating force through the pedals and you have the momentum of the pedals and apparatus itself, you are almost always going to get overshoot. The Schwinn Airdyne model, which has the arm levers attached, has a heavy momentum built into the pedals and is the very worst choice.

Creating a situation where overshoot is likely to occur is flat out stupid. Considering the options explained above, no wonder people have wildly different outcomes with range progression. We give them exercises where they have poor mechanical advantage or that can only be used in certain situations or where they are likely to overshoot and cause pain to themselves. I think we can do much better.

The other way I would like you to think about leverage is to regard the system in its entirety. It is a strategic advantage, or the power to act effectively. That is why there are seven silver bullets of success, not just one. Once you start putting the seven principles together you will see the power and effectiveness that is released. Do one or two of the seven principles only and you are likely to conclude that the fast track method does not work. Do all seven and you will absolutely kick a--.

Do you want to deal with a stiff knee for 6, 8 even 12 weeks, or do you want to knock out the range and thereby the pain medicine in a short but intense two-week period? Will you continue to be building basic and then functional strength beyond two weeks? Yes, but that is the easy part. It's your choice. Use the amazing leverage the system provides you, and put rehab in your rear view mirror.

LOW FRICTION

This has to be the most neglected of the seven silver bullets. I routinely use a firm slick board that the patient can use to slide his leg on when doing the bed program. If I don't have a board, I could use the backside of a new cookie or baking sheet. Most therapists don't see the value in this or view it as unnecessary. Why not just let them slide their leg on the sheets or a plastic bag?

Well, just a little something called "drag." State of the art bedding now includes pillow top mattresses, foam toppers and Tempurpedic memory foam (the worst thing devised yet for increasing the drag coefficient). A plastic bag is unacceptable because you still have the weight of the leg creating drag because the surface is not firm. There is also the problem of different types of flooring having drag, which is partially why the track was created.

"Drag" or friction sucks energy away from your desired goal, which is bending your knee effectively. That energy is required to overcome other random forces and cannot be regained. In other words, we are setting up a system where a good part of your effort is wasted. Why would I do that?

Call me insane, call me a perfectionist but I want every stroke that my patients take to give them the most return for their time and effort. If I lower drag and friction every heel slide, every sitting leg slide, every side-to-side motion on the bed gets a greater range of motion and psychologically is easier. Why would I not do this?

COMPLIANCE

Compliance is a term we therapists use to describe a patient's adherence to a prescribed program. It is an evaluative term looked at through our lens. Diligence, discipline or follow through would be the terms you would likely use in its place. Can you put this program into practice and grind it out? Will you put this program into practice and grind it out? What factors make it more likely than not that you will continue?

When I show people this system, typically on the first day that they are home from the hospital, I know that initially they may feel a little overwhelmed. Partially that is the timing. You the reader on the other hand are learning about this, hopefully before your surgery, and will be forewarned and forearmed. But after the patients realize the routine doesn't change much, especially the first two weeks, they settle in and can get down to business.

This program is methodical and perhaps tedious but the tradeoff is that it is highly effective and of relatively short duration (2-3wks to get the range) It is a highly leveraged system where one small piece makes the other small pieces go better. Perhaps the one thing that clinches it for people and seals their commitment is the feedback. They literally can see improvement as their toe inches backward on the Track and as the FLEX bar gets closer and closer to the edge of the chair. They realize... they are doing it; they are winning, they are feeling in command and in control of the situation, not wondering if their knee will come out right again, but just "when" it will be right.

The seven silver bullets help you the patient make quick work of your rehab time, wasting little or no effort, whereas your neighbors are battling back to baseline everyday, feeling confused, frustrated and wondering who they should trust. They will wish repeatedly that they would progress faster and not knowing better will have tapered off the pain medicine way too early, thinking that they will get addicted, and ruining their chances of a quick recovery.

This system has been proven successful across hundreds of different patients. You can see I have acted as a patient advocate in incorporating many of these bullets. I want you to have little or no pain, get off pain medicine quicker, get your range faster, use every ounce of energy expended purposefully and effectively and see measurable results along every step of the way!

"It's a no brainer, these principles not only make sense, they work!"

Pre-surgical Considerations

WHEN TO GIVE UP THE "OLD" JOINT?

The tipping point for each person is different. Age, medical condition, fear of doctors/ hospitals, pain tolerance, present activity levels, family support and assistance, present life circumstances and employment all play a role in influencing a decision for or against a total knee replacement. These are all very personal factors.

The question could be asked two different ways: "How much pain are you willing to tolerate to maintain your present activity levels?", or "How much activity are you willing to avoid and still consider your quality of life satisfactory?" An example is a 78-year-old woman who got her knee replaced because she could no longer enjoy biweekly roller-skating outings.

Most people over the age of 50 know at least 1-2 people who have had a total knee replacement whether it be parents, grandparents, in-laws, relatives, coworkers or just acquaintances. The outcomes of those surgeries will necessarily impact attitudes toward the surgery.

As this surgery has matured and become much more common, people generally have more favorable attitudes overall. It does not seem as much like a "crazy thing" to do...have your knee replaced.

Another newer trend is the somewhat cavalier attitude toward a knee replacement, as if one were doing something rather commonplace. Ten percent of adults in their 80's have had a knee replacement and 5% of adults over 50, but the data on how long a TKR will last in this younger group is non existent. We really do not know what the outcomes will be in a much younger, much more active population. Will this potentially necessitate more revision surgeries with potentially increased

33

complications? Will we as a country have the money to perform these at the pace we are performing them now? Don't get me wrong, it is an amazing surgery but people should think critically with wisdom when making this serious decision.

STRUCTURAL DEFORMITY

Another factor to consider from a Physical Therapy rehab perspective: Structural deformity in your knee prior to surgery makes the recovery process harder. A varus or a valgus knee commonly called bowlegs or knock-knees causes the soft tissues around your knee to accommodate to the increasing side bend in your knees. Once a knee is out of line, gravity acting on that knee will accelerate the process. The longer you wait the more things get out of line.

The knee can be straightened during surgery, but you will generally experience more discomfort in the soft tissues around the knee and sometimes even in the ankle in the recovery process.

ATROPHY AND RANGE OF MOTION

The other major factor is length of disability prior to surgery. Dragging, hopping, or limping on one leg for an extended period will cause atrophy or weakness of the muscles surrounding the joint and in the hip. When this happens it takes longer to build the muscle back up after surgery. The same can be said for range of motion deficits. People with pain tend to bend the knee less and therefore are susceptible to contractures prior to surgery. The longer range of motion has been limited, the longer and harder it is to get back.

BILATERAL VERSUS SINGLE TOTAL KNEE REPLACEMENT

As a physical therapist who has seen hundreds of total knee patients over many years, I would never recommend doing both knees at once if you can't tolerate pain medication, and generally I would caution against it because of the potentially greater risk of complications. Studies have shown that a bilateral total knee procedure puts the patient at...

Three times increased risk of death during the 30 days period for people > 70 years (Parvizi, 2001, Restrepo, 2007)

Twice increased risk of complication, especially vascular complications such as deep vein thrombosis (Ritter, 1997 Restrepo, 2007)

Much higher need (17 times) for banked blood with all possible complications (Lane, 1997)

Three times increased risk of cardiopulmonary complications; Twice increased length of the stay at the intensive unit department; Twice increased need for prolonged rehabilitation; Higher rate of bone marrow emboli into the brain (Sulek 1999)

However, another study by Bulluck et al., (2003) determined that rates of some peri-operative complications, including myocardial infarction, postoperative confusion, and the need for intensive monitoring, were greater after the bilateral arthroplasties. However, the thirty-day and one-year mortality rates and the risks of pulmonary embolism, infection, and deep venous thrombosis were similar for the two groups.

The conflicting outcomes of studies underlie the importance of the surgeon, I believe. Many patients successfully complete both knees at the same time. It requires going to a rehab facility following surgery and takes a special constitution to face the daunting tasks of doing rehabilitation for two total knee replacements simultaneously. However, if your life circumstance dictate or your mental frame of mind requires a one time only recovery, give it a try. Just remember to choose a very efficient surgeon with excellent technique. You are likely to be at higher risk for adverse events.

A CAUTIONARY TALE

The absolute worst outcome I have seen in all my years of therapy involved a bilateral knee replacement on a healthcare professional that was talked into doing the bilateral so that she would spend less time away from her practice. This individual suffered a nerve palsy on one leg from having the tourniquet applied too long and then got a bed sore that later became infected. If that wasn't bad enough the infection from the bed sore traveled to one of the knees. The result was that the patient had to undergo IV antibiotics and two more surgeries, one to remove the old total knee and place a spacer, and then another one to put in a new total knee.

That's bad but it gets worse. The knee got re infected and the same procedure of pulling the knee, IV antibiotics, and spacer placement had to be done again. This healthcare professional had spent 3 years dealing with this when I met her and she still had one more surgery to go to place the hopefully final knee.

I understand the natural inclination of people wanting to get the surgeries over with and get on with their lives and so they decide to get two done at once. However I believe that dealing with one at a time is the much more common sense way to proceed.

PARTIAL VS TOTAL KNEE REPLACEMENT

A partial knee replacement is just a method of fixing one side of the joint, usually the medial side instead of the entire joint that is done in a total knee replacement. There are plenty of sites on the web that describe both operations in detail so I won't go into that here.

The question I will delve into is, which one is better? On this topic there is significant controversy. Becker's Hospital Review has two articles that I highly recommend.

Are Partial Knee Replacements a Passing Trend or the Future of Knee Care?

13 Responses from joint replacement surgeons and industry experts (September 15, 2011)

http://www.beckersorthopedicandspine.com/sports-medicine/item/9290

Are Partial Knee Replacements a Viable Procedure?

15 Responses from orthopedic surgeons (September 22, 2011)

http://beckersorthopedicandspine.com/sports-medicine/item/9357

The clinical research is inconclusive, so that is why I am recommending reading the MD's opinions themselves. The following opinion from the second article summarizes my own very well.

Milton Smit, MD, OAK Orthopedics, Bradley, Ill.:

There's a high demand for uni-compartmental knee replacements, mainly because people perceive it is less surgery. A lot of physicians feel it has a higher function than total knee replacements, and sports medicine physicians generally have a higher interest in performing them than joint replacement surgeons. I've performed partial knee replacements, and I've found them more demanding than total knee replacements, and less forgiving. The alignment needs to be near perfect and it's harder to ensure the fixation is right. As a result, it is my perception that there is a higher failure rate among uni-compartmental knee replacements than total knee replacements.

The two procedures fail for different reasons. Total knee replacements fail because of infections or wear while uni-compartmental procedures can Sometimes, physicians say partials are easy to convert into revisions, but we have not found that true all of the time. In some case, there is bone loss and you have to implant long metal stems to make the procedure work. The polyethylene exchange in a total knee replacement is a much easier revision procedure. In my opinion, if you do a total knee, I think they last longer and are easier to revise.

In my experience, I have reached the same conclusion. The two most important factors include selecting the right patient and second, getting the alignment perfect. It is common sense if you think about it, that in combining a natural side with an artificial side, that you better get the alignment just right or you will actually cause increase wear on the natural side.

MakoPlasty, a robotic tool to assist in aligning the partial knee, has helped in this regard. Many people report very good outcomes with the increase precision of the partial alignment. Another consideration is the difficulty of a revision surgery of a partial to total knee replacement. While opinions vary, most will say it adds to the technical difficulty of the surgery.

Pearse et al. (2010), a study done in New Zealand, states that the rate of revision for the conversion of a partial to a total was four times higher than that for a primary TKR. They also stated that the rate of revision for conversion of a failed partial to another partial was 13 times higher than that for a primary TKR.

My summary includes the following if you want to follow the partial route:

1. Make sure you fit the characteristic of someone who would benefit, having only medial compartment damage.

2. Find a surgeon who has performed many partial surgeries, has been doing them for quite a long time, and has a high survival rating of 90% or higher for at least 7-10 years.

Survival rate is just the percentage of patients who have had the partial surgery and have the original components last for the years specified.

Avoid someone whose revision rate is high! The last thing you want to do is undergo a surgery you think will last and then in less than 2 years have to undergo a total knee replacement. Trust me I have talked to the patients themselves and they are very upset. They think their problems are solved; only to find out they really need the big one. Meanwhile their knee is now in worse shape having undergone this failed partial experiment.

REHABILITATION CENTER VERSUS HOME

Since I have worked the majority of my career as a home health physical therapist, I am naturally biased toward coming right home out of the hospital. The advantages are that you get away from a lot of germs that might be floating around a rehab place. All rehab places are not equal; some do a great job with infection control and others do not. Also there are many more people in a rehab center that could be carrying colds and flu with whom you might come in contact. When your resistances are low after surgery, it is a lot easier to pick up something, not to mention any infection in your knee, which you want to avoid at all costs.

When you go home, you go home to the things you are used to. And generally speaking you will be more active. I tease with my patients after they come out of rehab that they must have been at club med because they are behind in progress compared with most of my other patients who came directly home after the hospital.

The problem with rehab centers is that the PT sessions are only twice a day. This is too low a frequency (See section on the importance of frequency). Even with twice daily sessions much of it will not be in direct contact with a therapist. Usually there are multiple patients getting therapy at the same time and you will not always get the attention you need. In the home setting, it is one on one with the therapist for the entire time. You get live time correction if you are doing an exercise wrong or substituting the wrong muscle for a particular activity. Most rehab places hire the youngest or newest therapists, as well, so don't expect the most experienced folks.

The requirements for going home include being able to safely do the stairs into your home, being able to get in and out of bed safely and mobility with the walker. If you can do those three things you can go home. Most people think that they can't manage without a caregiver at home during the day. That is not true. It takes a little planning to think ahead about meals, having medicine handy, easy to use icing technique and where to do your exercises, but it can be done. In fact, it is done all the time by patients who prefer the comfort and familiarity of their own home.

I might add that having to wait for someone in a rehab place to take you to the bathroom drives independent souls crazy. Simply put you are not on your own schedule but theirs.

I would even suggest that you could still go home even if your bedroom is on the second floor. DME (Durable Medical Equipment) companies can deliver a hospital bed to set up downstairs for a few weeks to make things easier.

CHOOSING A REHAB CENTER

Despite my preference for starting your rehab at home, there is a time when that just is not possible. If that is the case for you, do your do diligence and examine each facility in more detail. As a home care therapist, I was always subjected to rants from patients who had recent bad experiences at the place they just left. I honestly don't know of one place locally that was not eventually a target of such a person who was really dissatisfied, despite the level of care they gave.

I think that some of the reasons for this is that younger patients are just running at a different speed and have very different expectations than your average 70 year old with multiple medical problems. I am saying this to qualify that any rehab place can be badmouthed, and listening to just word of mouth recommendations may not be the best way to pick your facility.

There is a much more objective way to evaluate facilities and that is the medicare.gov website that gives 5 star overall quality ratings for each facility based on the following criteria.

- Health inspections
- Nursing Home Staffing
- Quality Measures

It also includes the details for three other categories that are really important. These categories are...

- Fire Safety Inspections
- Penalties and Denials of Payment Against the Nursing Home
- Complaints and Incidents

A complaint is a problem reported by residents, their families, and nursing home staff. An incident is a problem reported by the nursing

40

home staff. Some complaints can lead to enforcement actions because the nursing home isn't complying with regulations.

It allows you to compare three facilities at a time side by side. You can find that information here:

http://goo.gl/bJmiVR

Unfortunately, you will not find any data on the therapy quality. As was mentioned earlier, these facilities tend to attract the young therapists for entry-level jobs, which is not necessarily a bad thing- energy and enthusiasm counts for a lot, but generally they are not the most experienced.

Another issue is the number of patients to therapist ratio, Typically a therapist is assigned a number of patients at the same time, meaning you don't get one on one care.

They set you up doing one exercise and then move over and get another patient going and come back to you later. So if you are not doing an exercise correctly it might not be noticed until later if at all. And if you are the type to slow down or quit when someone is not watching you'll have plenty of chance to attempt those maneuvers.

Many patients like the camaraderie that they can feel going through a similar difficult experience with someone else and generally that is a good thing. Ongoing friendships that offer mutual support and encouragement can be very beneficial throughout this whole process.

The social dynamics of comparison can work for or against you in such a setting. Those who see someone far ahead can get discouraged but on the other hand someone else might get more motivated to match the other persons success. So really it can cut both ways. Know yourself and what your tendencies are in social situations to make the best choice.

One more little pet peeve that I have to mention is the ridiculousness of having all the TKR patients participate in OT or occupational therapy. I think this is a big money maker that wastes your time and the governments' dollars. For the most part, if you have no upper extremity issues you do not need this. Of course, it never hurts to get rid of a little upper body flab but it is not really necessary. I would love to see two more PT sessions replacing these two semi-wasted sessions.

Something I am really sensitive to is not burning out your rehab motivation. People have only so much time and effort they want to devote to "getting over" their surgery. This is a limited quantity and I don't want to waste any of it on useless things.

The more I have you focus on random things the less focus you will be placing on the very important things. And believe me, there are some super important things early on that will make or break the length of the rehab process.

Is It Possible To Do A Knee Replacement Out Of Town?

If you happen to live in a rural area that is underserved by an outstanding orthopedic surgeon, by all means take the trip. When I was in Virginia Beach I did home care at an extended stay motel for a few people. In my experience, the best surgeons have a paternalistic attitude about the rehab and they watch over it carefully. For example, two of the surgeons I worked for would "fire" you from their patients if you did not do a good job. So if you go out of town to an excellent surgeon, chances are that you will get excellent rehab care as well.

SURGEON AND HOSPITAL SELECTION

Think body carpentry. Would you hire your next-door neighbor's sixteen-year-old son to reframe a doorway in your home? Or would you want to get an experienced carpenter of 20 years? Now I am not suggesting that some surgeons have the skills of sixteen year olds, but I am acknowledging the importance of experience and "practice."

To find a surgeon, I would look for the top three doctors in your local area in terms of volume. Those who do the surgery over and over and basically specialize in total joint replacement are better than the general orthopedic who sees any type of fracture or bone pathology.

A study of 80,904 Medicare patients noted that patients who had a first time total knee replacement done by surgeons who performed more than 50 procedures annually, had fewer complications than patients who had surgeons with an annual volume of 12 procedures or less (The Journal of Bone and Joint Surgery, 2004: 86; 1909-1916).

Pennsylvania has a great example of ways the government can assist you in being an informed consumer, using available data to guide you decision making process. http://www.phc4.org/hipknee/ This website allows potential patients to search by hospital and by surgeons (joint replacement specialties) to find out about complications rates and readmissions.

The other major consideration is that high volume hospitals are safer. People, systems, surgeons get better at what they practice over and over. All complication rates are lower at high volume hospitals.

In a 2011 study by Singh et al., hospital volume was categorized by annual performance of less than 25 surgeries, 26 to 100 surgeries, 101 to 200 surgeries (defined as low-volume hospitals), or greater than 200 surgeries (defined as high-volume hospitals). Patients who underwent primary total hip arthroplasty at low-volume hospitals were reported to be more likely to develop pulmonary embolism within 30 days postoperatively than those patients who underwent surgery at a high-volume hospital. Furthermore, 1-year mortality was higher for patients who underwent total hip replacement at low-volume hospitals.

Singh et al., determined that patients 65 years of age and older had significantly higher odds for 1-year mortality after undergoing total knee arthroplasty at low-volume hospitals when compared to the odds found in higher volume hospitals. Causes of complications at low-volume hospitals, the authors theorized, could be connected to hospital procedures, as well as perioperative and postoperative care processes.

Remember, you are looking for a great surgeon, not a friend or social acquaintance. I have had many people tell me poor bedside manner turns them off. Keep perspective, if the doctor is great at his profession you should not care how friendly he is. It might make your experience maybe a bit more pleasant, but overall you want a great knee outcome, not sweet memories.

I have also had folks say that when they visited a busy orthopedic who specialized in total joints that they felt like cattle. They were put off by the volume and complained that it seemed like a mill, very impersonal. Now I certainly don't want my surgery done by someone rushing to make money and pushing the numbers too high, with the end result that care is compromised. Keep in mind though that some of the best Docs have a defined system set up that can seem a bit impersonal but delivers great quality.

The best thing to do is to set up appointments with the top three Doctors in the area. Consider using some or all of the following questions to drill down to important information.

What type of total joint would you use and how is it placed (cemented vs. bone ingrowth)?

What is the failure rate on the particular model of total joint you would like to have placed in my knee/hip?

How long have you been using that model and why do you use it?

Do you have a system that your patients follow?

What is the complication rate for your surgeries, including infection, DVT's or device problem?

Do you like to send your patient's home or to rehab and what do you suggest for me?

It is also beneficial to talk to other local health care personnel, like nurses and physical therapists about their experiences with a particular doctor. And of course talk to former patients. There is nothing like a walking, talking, living, breathing testimony to any surgeon's work.

WHAT ABOUT THE IMPLANT ITSELF?

Direct to consumer total knee marketing is I think ultimately a negative force. It gets people focused on the wrong things. Read the small excerpt from Total Knee Arthroplasty: A guide to Get Better Performance, a book I purchased for approximately $200.00 and thank your lucky stars that you do not have to read and comprehend for a living.

By using the three accessible anatomical axes, the femoral and tibial components can be positioned so that the knee is in correct varus-valgus alignment throughout the flexion arc. The ligaments then can be balanced by determining which ligaments are contracted based on their function in flexion and extension. Simply stated, ligaments that attach to the femur on or near the epicondyles are effective both in flexion and extension and those that attach distant from the epicondylar axis are effective either in flexion or extension, but not in both positions. To extend this concept further, it can be stated that the portions of the ligament complexes that attach anteriorly in the epicondylar areas stabilize primarily in flexion, and those that attach posteriorly in the epicondylar areas stabilize primarily in extension. Ligaments that attach far posteriorly on the tibia are most effective in extension, and those attaching anteriorly are primarily tensioned in flexion. (p. 171)

Had enough yet? This is a book created for orthopedic surgeons. Trust me it gets way too complicated for the average untrained person. If you actually think you can wade through all the competing theories on types of implants, their design and pros and cons as they related to your particular knee-- you are crazy.

In addition, a lot of the stuff out there is hype. A great example is the so-called high flexion knee that was recent touted as the latest breakthrough component. Studies subsequently revealed only a 2-3 degree difference between more standard components.

My rules of thumb are these:

- Just like in car buying, don't buy a new model when they have made many changes. It's too early to know if there are going to be unforeseen problems.

- Work to get the best doctor... then trust him to make the right decision for your knee. Don't even listen to the hype.

The Fast Track System

THE NUMBER ONE GOAL

The number one goal following a total knee replacement is RANGE OF MOTION- getting your knee to move freely again without stiffening up and with the widest available range. This includes both bending the knee and straightening it fully. This is the most arduous task facing the patient after surgery. One of my patients effectively described the morning feeling as Groundhog Day, the movie with Bill Murray, where he wakes up in the same place everyday and life is at a standstill. The reason the knee feels so tight and stiff in the morning is that it has been dormant the entire night, generally 8-10 hours.

Simply put, your knee wants to move. If you could move your knee immediately post op and continuously thereafter the rehab would go easier. Of course that is not humanly possible but the next best thing is the phrase "early and often", or "move, move move-bend, bend, bend."

PIECE OF CAKE

Ok so that sounds easy. Just bend my knee. The problem is... it hurts AND it's swollen, meaning there is more fluid than normal sitting in the middle of your knee joint. Ah my friend, this is where all the difficulty comes in. Every bone in your body, every neural circuit, is telling you that you should WAIT until the swelling and pain subside and THEN bend the knee. This however is a trick. The knee says, "Please keep me bent at a nice 30 degree angle, like when you are seated on a recliner so that I can rest and recover and then I will work very hard for you later."

What the knee does not tell you is that your body is immediately trying to heal itself post op, and that means to tighten everything up, kind of like a house settling or concrete drying; it would prefer to see stability. The connective tissue surrounding your knee can form scars and adhesions that cause your knee to stay unnaturally tight with a restricted range of motion for the rest of your life.
Moving your knee early and often in the days following surgery acts like oil or a natural lubricant keeping those tissues supple until you get the

range of motion you desire or what is possible with the particular make of knee replacement that your Doctor has selected for you.

Another important point to remember is that while it seems rational that you should rest and let the swelling go down before trying to bend the knee, in reality, bending the knee acts as a physiological pump to push fluid out of your knee and into the tissues to be gotten rid of by the body. Bending hastens the reduction of pain and swelling in your knee. I know it seems incredibly counter intuitive, but it's true.

WHAT ABOUT THE PAIN

Ok, now that I have broken down all your rational and natural defenses to exercise and bending the knee when it is swollen, let's deal with the pain issue next. The total knee would be so easy...except for the pain. It is human nature to avoid pain especially pain above the 5 out of 10 threshold. (Zero is no pain and 10 is pain so bad you want to go back to the hospital).

When people ask, "Why does this hurt so badly?" I tell them if you saw the surgery instead of asking that question you would be asking, "How could completely taking apart my knee and putting it back together ever solve my pain problem?" The truth is the first two weeks are tough battling the pain. Your weapon is the narcotic pain medicine.

TOP FIVE REASONS
Why people don't want to take their medication:

#1. I don't want to become addicted

#2. I hate the way it makes me feel (dopey, sleepy)

#3. I hate the side effects (constipation, nausea)

#4. I don't need to take the medication when my knee doesn't hurt

#5. I am a Marine and don't feel that I should have to take any pain medication :)

Unfortunately quite a few people have an aversion to taking any narcotic, as well they should. What happens is that their post surgical goal becomes making it through the process taking the least amount of pain medicine possible. Now that absolutely conflicts with the PT's primary goal of getting your RANGE OF MOTION back.

The best way to prevent addiction is to jump into your rehab early, get serious and get your range of motion back moving your knee early and often. If you do that you should not need to continue on narcotic pain medicine for that knee. Movement is the best solution to long-range lingering pain problems. Limited movement will always lengthen the duration of recovery and that means staying on pain medicines for a longer period of time.

I will admit that there are unwelcome and bothersome side effects of taking pain medicine, but in reality these side effects are only TEMPORARY and most can be managed though various strategies whereas loss of range of motion will be permanent.

Roller coaster pain management is another strategy to avoid. This is the patient who only takes their pain medicine "when they need it". They alternate between feeling warm and cuddly and wanting to pull their hair out. When this patient takes enough medicine to get relief they decide not to take it again until the knee hurts. This is a very bad strategy. Once your kidneys clear the pain medicine from your system, there is nothing left to battle the pain. This can result in excruciating breakthrough pain and leads to incredibly inconsistent follow through with your exercise program because most people can NOT continue to bend and exercise consistently when they are experiencing pain greater than 5 out of 10, and sometimes it can take upwards of one half a day to start feeling good again. During that time your resolve and commitment to exercise will have been sorely tested.

THE KEY TO ACHIEVING THE NUMBER ONE GOAL-FREQUENCY

The easiest solution is The FLEX Bar, a reliable and simple tool that you can use when sitting upright in your favorite chair located in the "TV room" You do not need access to a staircase, a bed or a recliner. In fact you do not need to move away from the chair or the TV and therefore can be working on your range on and off all day.

The FLEX Bar greatly enhances compliance, makes you self determining and utilizes a biomechanical advantage to overcome the stiffness and tightness you feel in your post surgical knee. Stretching frequently allows you to maximize your efforts. Consider the following chart.

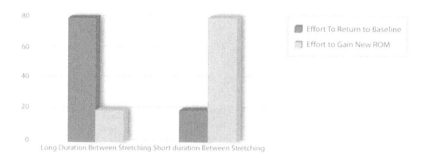

Baseline is any patient's previous maximum range of motion. When a patient takes a long break between stretching, they will spend most of their next exercise effort regaining motion that they have lost or battling back to the baseline. This is wasted effort. If they return to stretching exercises sooner, they will spend only a minimal effort battling back to the baseline and most of their effort will go into gaining new range of motion for that session. This is one of the most important keys to gaining back ROM.

A WORD ABOUT THE CPM MACHINE

CPM stands for Continuous Passive Motion. The tool was designed to keep the patient's knee moving early in the rehabilitation process so that scar tissue could not form. They were readily adopted after initial studies showed that people who used CPM machines did better than their counterparts. Later on however, conflicting studies clouded the clear support for CPM machines. Today in the United States, the CPM is most times used prior to discharge from the hospital, and is used maybe 50% of the time in a patient's home.

Your physician may or may not order a CPM. I like to think of it like this. If you do get one it is a bonus if you don't rely on it exclusively; and if you don't get one, no worries, you will do just fine. I see it all the time. The Fast Track program is based on similar principles of frequent leveraged exercise as that of the CPM, except that you are using your arms and our Flex Bar tool for the leverage. So what's the difference? When you actively flex your knee you are much more engaged in the process, you can get in a higher number of repetitions in less amount of time, you are sitting upright which is a big benefit to you from a cardiovascular stand point (heart does not get weaker), and you can be located in any room in the house. For all of these reasons you have more flexibility and control of the rehab process.

STRETCHING INTENSITY

Learning the proper intensity with which to stretch the knee is very important! I like to divide the different intensity levels into three parts.

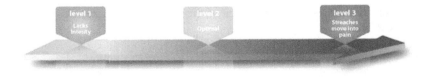

A **level one** stretch is a low intensity stretch. It is a relatively easy motion that will only maintain your present range. Generally you are able to do other activities as well, like talk on the phone, watch TV or read the newspaper. Your progress with range of motion will be minimal or non-existent. There is a high potential to form adhesions.

A level three stretch is a high intensity stretch. You are trying to move too fast in the rehab process; to stretch too far in one movement from where you were previously. This is why it is important to measure your knee progress. This stretch will usually cause pain and a reflexive withdrawal of the motion. It may even result in you having to take a day or two off from rehab to give time for your knee to recover.

Basically this approach is counter-productive even though it might seem that you are working really hard. Also you may become gun shy about bending if you constantly put yourself in this situation. It may also result in you being less compliant with the exercises because it is hard to beat yourself up on a regular basis.

A level two stretch is a moderate intensity stretch. There will be some discomfort and pulling feeling in your knee. You will want to count how many you are doing because it will not seem easy, but it is manageable with good pain management. When a patient is in this mode they are focused and do not want to chitchat or do anything else while so engaged.

When my patients are working at this level 4 times a day they gain 2-3 new degrees of range of motion a day. When looked at in the perspective of one day, this seems discouraging; however, the total improvement for one week would be 14-21 degrees, and for two weeks 28-42 degrees. Like I said earlier, most people can gain the majority of their range back in the first two weeks. At this point, you can then start to taper down your pain medicine and get back to feeling "normal".

The Fast Track Total Knee Program– Featuring The FLEX Bar

Exercises are to be completed at least four times a day. If you want to do more you will be rewarded. The reason for this is that your leg wants to move. If you do a set at 9 am, 1 p.m., 4 p.m., and 7 p.m., you are moving your leg every 3-4 hours throughout the day. This keeps your knee loose. The worst set will be in the morning because your knee has been dormant all night. It seems as though you are starting at ground zero but just keep at it in about 2 weeks you will have most of your knee range back.

BED EXERCISES: WARM-UPS

Ankle Pumps-Pull toes toward head of the bed flexing both ankles simultaneously then point them away toward the foot of the bed (2 sets of 10 gradually advancing to 1 set of 25-30)

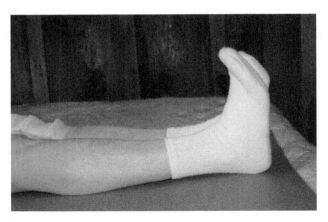

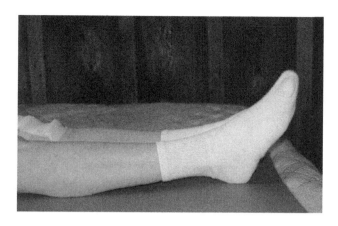

Knee Squeezes- Place towel roll under knees and then push down into the roll, then relax. I like patients to push firmly and generate some force but I do not have my patients hold for five seconds. You can do this lying down but if you have any difficulty figuring out what you are supposed to be doing, sit up and attempt the exercises from the long sitting position (see picture). There are other muscles of the hip that you could use to substitute movement for the quad muscles (directly on top of your thigh) when lying down, sitting up will force you to perform the exercise correctly. Your quads will be the only muscle that can perform the movement in this position. (2 sets of 10 gradually advancing to 1 set of 25-30)

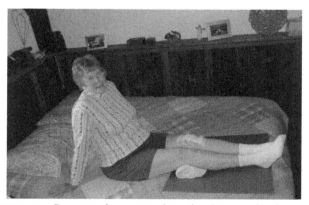

Butt Squeezes- Squeeze butt muscles simultaneously then relax. No picture you have to envision this one yourself:) (2 sets of 10 gradually advancing to 1 set of 25-30)

55

Heel Slides-Slide heels on board toward your bottom, (Do not worry about getting maximal range, just move the leg back and forth without resting at either end of motion) (2 sets of 10 gradually advancing to 1 set of 25-30)

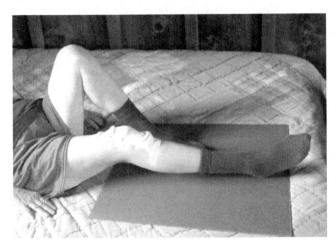

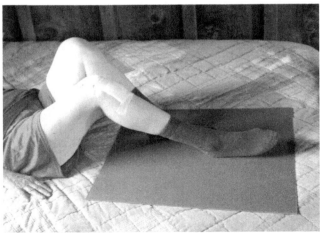

Windshield Wipers- Slide leg side to side on board keeping ankle flexed toward your head and foot perpendicular to the ceiling. Do not rest on either end of the side-to-side motion. (2 sets of 10 gradually advancing to 1 set of 25-30)

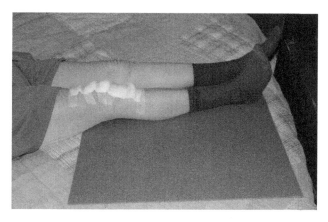

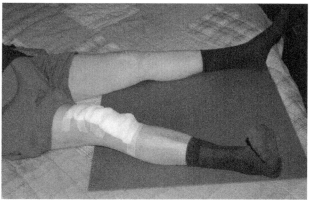

QUAD WORK

Straight Leg Raises-Bend opposite leg first. Get assistance to lift affected leg into high starting position (If your hamstrings are tight, you will only be able to get to 45 degrees, but if they are loose, some people, especially women, can lift leg to almost 90 degrees.)

"Higher and faster" is easier--"Lower and slower" is harder in this exercise. Start with 4 sets of 5 moving the leg downward from starting position about 12" and then back up. Rest after the 5th one. Repeat 4 times. Your exercise helper will spot your leg making sure that you are safe.

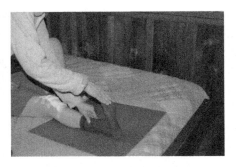

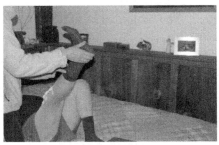

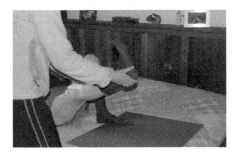

Leg kicks-sitting on the side of the bed. Put towel under thigh of affected leg. Straighten leg as much as possible. Do 2 sets of 10 progressing to 20-25 repetitions.

Knee to chest- Advanced exercise- only do when your therapist tells you it is appropriate. Keep opposite knee bent. Lift affected leg bringing your knee toward your chest as high as you can go, straighten leg out again fully. Do two to three sets of 5 to start. These are hard. Go easy at the beginning. Start with 5 repetitions then increase.

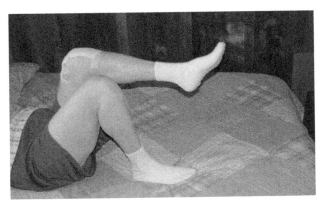

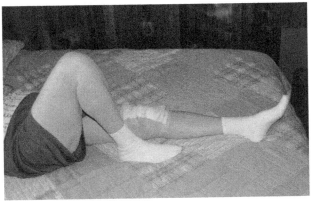

CHAIR EXERCISES- THE TRACK

Single Leg Slides- Using The FLEX Track slide your affected leg back and forward in a set of 10 reps holding the last rep approximately 10-15 seconds.

Do not slide your leg very far forward, as this decreases backward thrust. Focus on the backward motion.

Do 3 sets of 10 at or beyond your previous mark on The FLEX Track. This will ensure that you are making progress. This may mean that you do 3 sets of 10 to get back to your old mark and another 3 sets of 10 beyond the new mark.

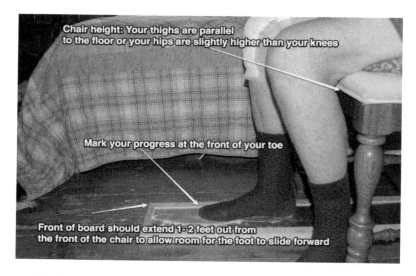

Chair height: Your thighs are parallel to the floor or your hips are slightly higher than your knees

Mark your progress at the front of your toe

Front of board should extend 1-2 feet out from the front of the chair to allow room for the foot to slide forward

Double Leg Slides-Place good leg over affected leg at the ankle. Use good leg to assist affected leg in pulling back (Sometimes your surgical leg is weak coming into the surgery and can use a little help)

Forward Slide in Chair-Place affected leg as far back as is comfortable. Using armrest, lift your body up just slightly and slide forward about one inch. This should stretch your knee slightly. Hold for 10-15 seconds. Take a deep breath, relax into the stretch, and then repeat by moving forward another one inch, relaxing and holding for 10-15 seconds. Repeat one more time, and then slide all the way back.

CHAIR EXERCISES- THE FLEX BAR

The FLEX Bar-The Flex Bar will help you successfully rehabilitate your new total knee by using a simple but effective bio-mechanical advantage to stretch your swollen and stiff post surgical knee and can be easily stored close by you to ensure compliance to the high frequency stretching that maximizes effort and minimizes wasted time.

Place the ball of your foot, not the arch, on the bar in the middle of The FLEX Bar. Place both hands on the topsides of the bar and slowly pull the bar toward your knee until you feel your knee stretching at a #2 level (explained below). If you can pull the bar to your knee without too much discomfort "walk" the legs of the Flex Bar closer to your body by lifting one leg of the FLEX bar, placing it approximately 1 inch closer to you on the floor and then lifting the opposite leg of the FLEX bar and placing it in the same manner. Do another set of 10 at this level and hold the last rep for 10-15 seconds. Release the stretch. If this stretch seemed hard (level 3 stretch) repeat another set of 10 at this level.

If it seems like you can do more, advance the FLEX bar closer to you and repeat another set of 10 pulling the bar to your knee. Hold the stretch again. Motion can be seen in the following three photos.

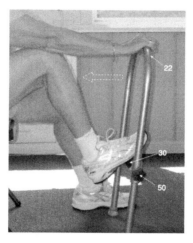

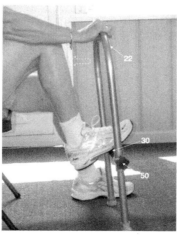

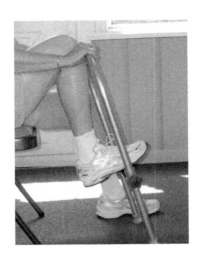

CHAIR TO CHAIR HANG- EXTENSION

Chair-to-Chair Hang- Place a wooden chair with a rolled up towel on it in front of you. Lift your surgical leg and place your ankle over the towel roll. Your surgical leg should be suspended between to the two chairs causing a stretch to the back of the knee. Maintain this position for two minutes. (If you have severe pain, you can hold for less.) Continue to build up your time until you can "hang" for 5 minutes. After you start tolerating the "hang" you will add the following during the 2-5 min session:

*Add Quad sets- Activate the muscle on top of your thigh helping to drive your knee straight. Do 1-2 sets of 10

*Add Hamstring stretch-Lean forward and stretch your hand toward your lower calf or foot if possible hold for 10-second count and repeat 5-7 times. Remember to breath, this relaxes your muscles.

*Add Weight to the Chair Hang- Add weight after you can tolerate the chair hang for 5 minutes. Take two plastic food bags and tie the ends together. Put a can in each bag and drape it over your knee, being careful to keep the ends off your incision line for increase comfort. Start by hanging the leg for **ONLY TWO** minutes, building back up again to 5 minutes. In time you will have most or all of your extension back.

Remember to actual time this stretch. Don't just ball park it. This is especially important if you had trouble straightening your leg prior to surgery. If you keep the leg up too long you might not be aware that you are over stretching your tendons. When you over stretch, you may experience lingering pain that will result in you having to omit the exercise for a few days, slowing down your progress. So remember don't overdo it. Better to go slow at first then be more aggressive when you know that your knee can tolerate it.

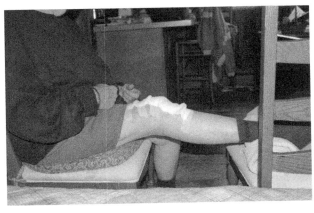

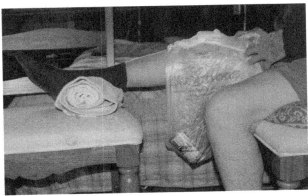

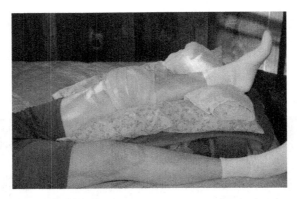

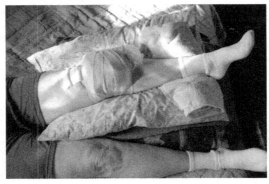

ICING TECHNIQUE

Elevate your surgical leg on pillows, foam, sofa cushion or big comforters to ensure a 30-degree angle of the leg in relation to the bed. You want the fluid to drain down to the heart. Your trunk should be relatively flat.

If you have trouble breathing when flat, you must elevate the trunk to be comfortable.

Compress the ice to the knee with an ace wrap or elastic bandage if available. Use crushed ice or one of the commercially available gel ice bags. You can also use a frozen bag of corn or peas but these will not be as cold. They can be reused for a couple of days for icing purposes, then discard.

REMEMBER THIS PHRASE : EARLY, OFTEN, EASY AND EFFECTIVE

The Fast Track Total Knee System has been designed to make you successful in transforming your surgical knee into your active DO-anything knee.

Easy and effective applies to how the Fast Track Total Knee system will assist you. The Track allows you to bend on the easy glide surface and to monitor and mark measurable progress. The FLEX bar makes bending your knee much easier and more effective with a biomechanical advantage. Both of these tools will help you achieve the goal of a pain free knee.

Early and often applies to your job in rehabbing your total knee. I recommend doing your exercises 4 times a day but don't let that limit you. Anytime you feel your knee stiffing up, go ahead and get on the FLEX bar and loosen up or jump on the track and start doing some more bending. It doesn't have to be a big session, just get loose again. These tools were designed to be portable, making it easy to do your rehab in the comfort of your own home in any room you prefer. Hang your leg into extension for short periods when you are watching TV then rest and walk around the house. Before you know it, you will start seeing amazing progress and you will feel better and better each day.

The Fast Track System on a Budget

How to make your own tools on the cheap

Everyone needs to save money these days, that's why I've included this chapter. I know that insurance deductibles and co-pays are going up all the time, and if you can find a way to do this cheaply and effectively, my guess is that you'll be all in. There are three essential tools that you need to have. You have heard me discuss them in the previous chapters; the slider for the bed, The Track, and the FLEX bar. Let me give you a cost effective way to secure each one of these tools or an effective substitute.

THE SLIDER

As I mentioned previously, what is needed is a firm low friction surface on which you can glide your foot and leg, while positioned on the bed. I have used a piece of Masonite cut into a 2 x 2 square. Masonite is found at your local Lowes or Home Depot and usually comes in a 4'x 8' sheets for about 10-12 bucks. I have a worker from Lowes cut the sheet up into 8 squares. It works great for me, I get a bunch of squares that I can now use with patients that I throw in the back of my car. You, of course, don't need 8 - 2'x 2' squares, so if you know someone handy who can cut up a 2' x 2' piece of Masonite, Plexiglas or white board, that would work fine as well.

Another common household item that you could use is a cookie sheet or baking sheet, new or only slightly used for lower friction. The large flat kind with only one edge works the best and gives you the largest surface area with which to do the exercises. I've known people who have bought these at the dollar stores for next to nothing. If you use the cookie sheet option you will most likely have to change the orientation of the sheet to get maximal range in two different directions. The heel slide is a long slide on a line toward your body and the windshield wipers is a long slide in a side-to-side direction to get yourself the greatest range. This can be slightly difficult to do if you are alone and just starting out. This is why the Masonite piece is the best option but the cookie sheet works all the time but takes a bit of effort to change the orientation of the sheet.

THE TRACK

The track is the piece of equipment on which you slide your foot back and forth, trying to maximize range. Actually you don't need a track if you have a very low friction surface at home that is out of the way of foot traffic where a chair can be placed up against a wall for the duration of approximately 2-3 weeks.

A strip of masking tape or painters tape can be laid down perpendicular to the wall that the chair is positioned against to mark progress. If the thought of putting any kind of tape down on your floor makes you faint, then secure a yardstick perpendicular to the wall and mark your progress on that. If the yardstick does not come out far enough away from the wall then simply place an object like a book or an old VCR tape between it and the wall making it come out further in front of the chair. You could also position the yard stick where you want it (it should come out in front of the chair far enough for you to be able to measure the front of your toe- approximately 1-2 feet), then put a mark on the yardstick at the level of one of the chair legs and make sure the yardstick is always lined up with that mark.

I personally like to be able to push the yardstick up against something and leave it there. When you have to line the mark up with the chair leg it can get shifted around or moved unbeknownst to the patient, then they came back some time later and they are upset because they think they lost 2 inches of range. Bottom line is either way works. Do what is best for you and your situation.

If overall a stationary chair atop low friction flooring is not going to work for you given your household set up, then you should try to make a track which you can use in any part of the house. The track can consist of Masonite, white board or any low friction surface. You could mark directly on the board or place a yardstick near or on top of the board to track your progress.

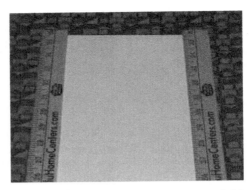

Here is a picture of a piece of white board 6" by 36" with two yardsticks glued onto the edges

Below is a picture of the backside of the Track. I have glued some shelf liner to the back to make it non- skid. Shelf liner is available at Lowes or you may have some leftovers stuck in a drawer somewhere. At any rate, it is not expensive and recommended if you are going to be doing your slides on any surface where the track may move about as you attempt to use it. You might be able to get away without any backing if you will be working on a thick carpet.

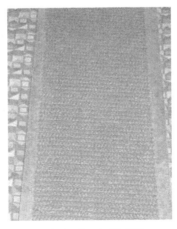

Backside of Homemade Track unit (Shelf liner on white board)

THE FLEX BAR

The easiest way to make a low budget FLEX bar is to find an old standard walker. A standard walker is one with four rubber tip feet. You do not want a walker with wheels. You need the rubber tips to keep the tool from sliding away from you. Finding a walker is not too hard. Lots of community groups have an assortment of old walkers. Friends, aunts, uncles, in short anyone who you know who has had surgery might have one collecting dust in a closet somewhere. One thing to note however is that Medicare will only purchase one walker in a five-year period for a person. So if you know that someone might need that walker again, best not to use. You can find them at garage sales or on Craig's list. Many people have durable medical equipment that is in good condition that they want to get rid of after someone they know passes away.

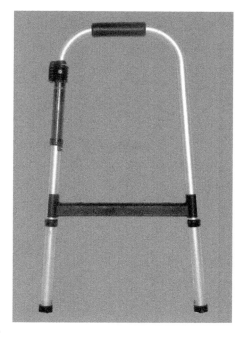

Once you have found your walker, you need to find someone with a hacksaw or saw that can cut through metal and you are going to cut off the side of the walker. Once that is done file down the rough edges and then tape over the hole and edging with duct tape or foam or something that will ensure that no one will cut themselves in handling the tool.

If you want to get a little fancy, take some non-skid flooring strips and put them on the bar in the center to help hold your foot into position on the circular bar, and that's it! You have a functional FLEX bar that will help you accomplish your goals.

Another slightly more complicated way to get your own FLEX Bar is to construct one out of PVC pipe. Stay with me until the end of the book and I will let you know how you can get the blueprints to create your own. Really this is very simple to do as well.

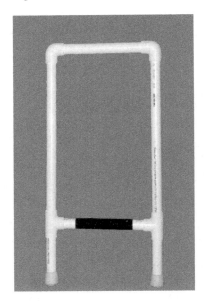

The Fast Track System Integrated

How to work this out within the current medical system

This is the trickiest part of attempting to promote this method to the masses. You will all be working with another therapist who may or may not value what I have to say. So why did I do it this way you might ask? Simply stated, if something works and is helping people I think they should have access to it quickly. This system has been fully vetted. When I say vetted I do not mean research.

The principles in this system have been researched exhaustively in many other disciplines. It stands as common knowledge in fitness literature, business literature, sports and performance literature, weight lost literature, that measurable feedback systems help people monitor and improve their performance. It is common sense to believe that low friction surfaces post surgically will not only encourage you by making your routine as easy as possible, it will also maximize all your efforts. We already use leverage in our total knee rehab, so the FLEX bar is simply an easier, portable tool to help you capitalize on that leverage. The frequency of exercises was given to me by fiat from a pioneer in total knee surgeries, Dr. Louis Jordan, in the early 90's. I certainly wouldn't be one to say that just because a physician said it, it was the gospel truth, but I have worked with this method for over 20 years now and know from an experiential standpoint that it works.

So did I want to waste three to five years on a research project before getting this out to you, the end user. A solid "Hell no" is the answer! In a sense you are participating in the new Internet revolution that explodes our ability to distribute ideas of any kind to huge numbers of people. The traditional gatekeepers have been thrown out of the tower, so to speak. Health care will be affected as everything else is affected.

As I said earlier, a third party system does not exist to solely benefit the patient. If it did we would see more innovations because people who pay would demand it. Should we have better total knee rehab right now? Yes, but the people that could create it (the healthcare professionals) are all getting paid by the system already and don't stand to get paid anymore if they create something better. And to be honest for someone like me to try to manage all aspects of inventing, manufacturing and marketing while working at my current job is darn near impossible.

The approach that I believe is the most beneficial is to attempt to inform and engage the therapist who is assigned to you. The following is an open letter to my PT colleagues that you can have your physical therapist read.

Dear fellow PT:

Your patient has heard about the Fast Track system and wants to give it a try. I am a Home health PT of 20 years and have been developing this system along the way. I ask you to review the principles upon which this system is based, and I believe you will find them irrefutable. They simply make sense. They can be found in the chapter entitled, "The Seven Silver Bullets of Success". If you find the principles compelling, begin to use them in aggregate and you will see their power. If you have any questions or have valuable feedback feel free to contact me personally at michelle@totalkneereplacmentrecovery.net to discuss things further.

First and foremost, I take a focused minimalist approach to gaining range. You can work with your patient and not against them by limiting the number of exercises prescribed within the first two-three week period. Patients love to be distracted by other easier exercises than range development. Less really is more at the beginning. The more focused the patient is on range building, the easier and easier it gets. Once your patient has gained 120 degrees range of motion and has achieved a base level of strength more can be added. It really does work.

Yours in Therapy, Michelle Stiles

Show them the chapter on the principles, or better yet, steer them to purchase the book itself where they will have the fullest treatment to date of my system laid out for them. But even after this exchange you might find yourself working with someone who is just not open to receiving new ideas. You have two options. Throw my stuff by the wayside and engage with the therapist, or request a change of therapist. I would not recommend working at odds with the person assigned to you. It's too stressful in an already stressful time. If you know, like and trust the therapist assigned, by all means keep them.

I have to mention again why home care should be the desired setting for your immediate post-surgical rehab. In sub-acute rehab centers, you will waste tons of time doing occupational therapy exercises that you really don't need unless you have something specifically wrong with your arms, and your knee bending frequency will only be twice a day. You limit your flexibility to be captain of your own ship and of course you cannot bring homemade tools for your personal use even if you have good rationale because anything out of the ordinary just won't go over well.

While this isn't the straightest, easiest path that could be laid out for you, it may be the fastest route to getting a general widespread adoption of these methods.

By writing this book and you reading it, I am appealing directly to you the customer and the one on which these principles will have the most profound effect. I am content to let you be the judge and jury on these methods because with that big swollen knee perched in the middle of your leg looking completely daunting, you will be the one to know very quickly if what I am telling you works. No one else has such a compelling motivation staring them in the face. You then become the living breathing success story.

We also are taking advantage of the phenomenon called viral transmission. If something is good you can tell your friends and neighbors and they in turn can tell others. This is significantly more powerful than one article published in a journal that may or may not emerge into the general consciousness.

Big Trends

Food for Thought

In this final chapter I want to make you aware of some trends that are critically important and concern much more weightier issues than just the rehab aspect of the total knee replacement but looks at the surgery from a broad societal perspective.

Consider this quote taken from the background data informing a recent study by Ivan et al., in 2012, representing a consortium of healthcare systems including the Cleveland Clinic. This study examined administrative-level data for 10,910 people who had single leg total knee replacement surgery for a period for January 1, 2008 to 2009.

First, knee osteoarthritis is a common condition whose treatment is expensive. The lifetime risk of symptomatic knee osteoarthritis is estimated to be nearly 50 percent, and the two major risk factors are aging and obesity. In 2008, total knee replacement inpatient costs exceeded $9 billion—the highest aggregate cost among the ten procedures for which demand is growing the fastest. Between 2005 and 2030, the demand for primary knee arthroplasty in the United States is projected to grow by 673 percent, or 3.48 million procedures annually. More resource-intensive total knee revisions—a procedure that repairs or replaces a previous replacement—are projected to grow by 601 per- cent between 2005 and 2030. In 2005, medical expenditures for the treatment of arthritis were $353 billion, and they are expected to rise because of increases in the number of people with osteoarthritis. (p.2)

Do the math. Inpatient costs exceeded $9 billion in 2008 with approximately one-half million procedures or less performed, and the current estimate for procedures needed in 2030 is 3.48 million. We are headed straight into a crisis. More people are going to want and need this surgery than can be reasonably paid for by other members of society, namely the young and working. Also many will be unable to pay for the surgery themselves, the average cost being around 30-40K. The future burden we are creating is staggering. This trend is being accelerated by growing obesity rates among youth and the increasing propensity to offer knee replacements in the under 50 crowd.

Secondly, physicians who perform total knee replacements have had their Medicare reimbursement rates drop 36% from 1991 to 2006 with the average reimbursement being $1,442.

In contrast, hospital payments increased 19% and medical devices list prices and selling prices have increased 171% and 117% respectively from the same period. I personally know physicians who are frustrated over these financial arrangements. Frustrated physicians are not necessarily promoting the field to their sons and daughters. As the population ages, Medicare reimbursements will be largely dictating salaries. These events could cause the best and the brightest to steer away from medicine and toward more lucrative careers.

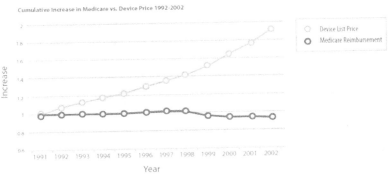

Medicare Reimbursement vs. Devise List Price from 1992-2002

Medicare Reimbursement vs. Devise List Price from 1992-2002

This data was complied by Healthpoint Capital Research in 2003 and is slightly dated but it is extremely difficult to get current information on these topics. For example, medical device companies frequently enact purchase agreements with confidentiality clauses so that hospitals cannot reveal the price paid for specific implants.

Senators Grassley and Spector introduced legislation in 2007 requiring disclosure of pricing by medical device companies. While I am not exactly sure what happened to torpedo this legislation, concerns over this issue have not abated. The quote below comes from the concluding section of a study done by the Government Accountability Office in 2012 entitled "Lack of Price Transparency May Hamper Hospitals Ability to Be Prudent Purchasers of Implantable Medical Devices." Total knee components fall under the heading of implantable Medical Devices or IMD'S.

The lack of price transparency for the IMDs we examined makes it difficult to know whether hospitals are achieving the best device prices. This lack of price transparency may have implications for Medicare because excess or unnecessary IMD costs that hospitals incur may be passed onto the Medicare program. In 2009, Medicare spent over $19 billion for hospital procedures involving IMDs. A substantial portion of this amount may be attributable to the cost of the devices themselves, but exactly how much is unknown, in part, because hospitals purchase the IMDs and Medicare does not track IMD prices or how much individual hospitals will pay for them.

Although Medicare's payment approach provides hospitals with an incentive to seek the best price on IMDs, hospitals may vary in their ability to achieve the best price because of limited price information and bargaining power. While we were able to obtain detailed IMD pricing data from 31 of the 60 hospitals we contacted, the effort revealed the challenges in compiling and analyzing meaningful price information even from this relatively small number of hospitals. Furthermore, we observed substantial variation in the prices that these 31 hospitals paid for cardiac devices.

Some hospitals paid several thousand dollars more than other hospitals paid for the exact same device produced by the same manufacturer. These data suggest that some hospitals have substantially less bargaining power with the small group of companies that manufacture particular IMD devices and consequently face challenges in obtaining more favorable prices.

Physician preferences for particular manufacturer's devices and models may further complicate hospitals' bargaining power. Such preferences may shape hospitals' purchasing decisions and limit their ability to obtain volume discounts from device manufacturers. Moreover, many device manufacturers require confidentiality clauses that prohibit hospitals from disclosing their negotiated prices with third parties, which may include physicians.

A hospital that is constrained in sharing price data with its physicians loses an opportunity to enlist their assistance in the hospital's efforts to be a prudent purchaser of IMD. (p. 29-30)

Putting the trends together, increasing numbers of people needing the surgery, decreasing physician reimbursements, increasing implant reimbursements, and decreasing hospital margins doesn't sound like a winning formula. Combine these factors with the general economic situation and the demographic trends of aging population in America and we are going to be facing many more tough choices in the future. These are the types of facts, which most Americans are unfamiliar, when discussing the future of healthcare in America.

Total knee replacement surgery is an amazing medical contribution to society with incredible success rate for eliminating pain in the knee caused by osteoarthritis. I've witnessed first hand, the transformation of a life once limited by pain now free to move with ease. I hope that this type of surgery will continue to be readily available to the general population and I hope that the contents of this book will have made it profoundly easier to navigate the post surgical rehab with minimal pain, pain medicine, effort and time sacrificed from more productive pursuits.

Final Thoughts

I hope you have enjoyed this ride exploring the total knee rehab journey from plenty of different perspectives and angles as much as I did. I hope as well that you now have total confidence and little fear of what the post surgical rehab process entails. Go back and reread the section on the seven bullets of success to seal those concepts in your mind. If you understand those, you are golden.

The first one to two days in the learning process will be the toughest but once you "get it" and begin to see the steady progress, it is just a matter of grinding it out and being diligent for about 1.5 to 2 weeks until you bag the coveted 120 degrees range of motion early in the sequence. Then you can kiss goodbye to the toughest part of the rehab, to the pain medicine, to constipation and to the 4 per day sessions. You now have another 3-4 weeks to get your strength back throughout the range, increase your walking distances and naturally regain your normal gait pattern.

References

American Physical Therapy Association. (2010). Joint Arthroplasty: Advances in Surgical Management and Rehabilitation. La Crosse, WI: Hughes.

Bellemans J, Rees MD, & Victor MK. (EDs.). (2005). Total Knee Arthroplasty: A Guide to Get Better Performance. Heidelberg, Germany: Springer.

Bullock, DP, et al."Comparison of Simultaneous Bilateral with Unilateral Total Knee Arthroplasty in Terms of Perioperative Complications" J. Bone Joint Surg. Am., Oct 2003; 85: 1981 - 1986.

Government Accountability Office. (2012). Lack of Price Transparency May Hamper Hospitals' Ability to Be Prudent Purchasers of Implantable Medical Devices (GAO-12-126). Washington, DC: U.S. Government Printing Office.

Ivan M. Tomek, Allison L. Sabel, Mark I. Froimson, George Muschler, David S. Jevsevar, Karl M. Koenig, David G. Lewallen, James M. Naessens, Lucy A. Savitz, James L. Westrich, William B. Weeks and James N. Weinstein A Collaborative Of Leading Health Systems Finds Wide Variations In Total Knee Replacement Delivery And Takes Steps To Improve Value. Health Affairs, , no. (2012): (published online May 9, 2012; 10.1377hlthaff.2011.0935)

Healthpoint Capital Research. "Merrill turns bearish on Orthopedics while Stephens puts its money into a sparkling Gem of a spine center. Guess who we think is the smarter investor!" April 7, 2003. Original Source: The Future of Orthopedics: Large Joint Reconstruction, Robin R. Young, John J. Chopack, Jr. 2003. Graph is of data from Table 3.8.

Lane GJ, Hozack, WJ, Shah S, et al. Simultaneous bilateral versus unilateral total knee arthroplasty:outcomes analysis. Clin Orthop 1997;345:106–12.

Miller L. (September 15, 2011) Partial Knee Replacements a Passing Trend or the Future of Knee Care?13 Responses Becker's Hospital Review. Retrieved from http://beckersortopedicandspine.com/sports-medicine/item/9290.

Miller L. (September 22, 2011) Are Partial Knee Replacements a Viable Procedure? 15 Responses. Becker's Hospital Review. Retrieved from http://beckersorthopedicandspine.com/sports-medicine/item/9357.

Mitzner RL, Petterson SC, Snyder-Mackler L. Quadriceps strength and the time course of functional recovery after total knee arthroplasty. J Orthop Sports Phys Ther. 2005; 35(7): 424-436.

Parvizi J, Sullivan TA, Trousdale RT, Lewallen DG: Thirty –Day Mortality Following Total Knee Arthroplasty. J. Bone Joint Surg. 83(A): 1157-61, 2001.

Pearse AJ, Hooper GJ, Rothwell A, Frampton C. Survival and functional outcome after revision of a unicompartmental to a total knee replacement: the New Zealand National Joint Registry. J Bone Joint Surg Br. 2010 Apr; 92:508-12

Ritter M, Mamlin LA, Melfi CA, et al. Outcome implications for the timing of bilateral total knee arthroplasties. Clin Orthop 1997;345:99-105

Restrepo C, Parvizi J, Dietrich T, Einhorn TA: Safety of simultaneous bilateral total knee arthroplasty: A meta-analysis. J Bone Joint Surg Am 2007; 89:1220–6

Singh JA, Kwoh CK, Boudreau RM, et al. Hospital volume and surgical outcomes after elective hip/knee arthroplasty: A risk adjusted analysis of a large regional database. Arthritis Rheum. 2011 Jun 7. doi: 10.1002/art.30390.

Sulek CA, Davies LK, Enneking FK, Gearen PA, Lobato EB. Anesthesiology. 1999;91(3):672-6.

As my way of thanking you for purchasing my book... I'd like to give you

4 FREE BONUSES
to help make your recovery even easier.

›› Quickie Exercise Sheet

Have the basic core group of exercises at your fingertips in a two page sheet. No need to flip back through a book or try to find something in a kindle version. It's your very own handy reference that you can keep with you and refer back to until you have the exercises down pat.

›› Daily Progress Tracker

Tracking your progress is invaluable. Now you can easily record and visualize the progress you are making session by session toward your recovery.

›› FLEX BAR Blueprint

Make your own personal version of the patented FLEX BAR at home in less than 30 minutes. Get a downloadable PDF file that shows you how to make a PVC substitute, that is very cost effective and simple to assemble.

›› Knee Recovery Leverage Analysis Tool

Take this short test to determine if your upcoming rehabilitation experience will be max-imized to include every available good practice. In some cases you might not know the answer to a question and this would be a good occasion to discuss the recovery sequence with your surgeon.

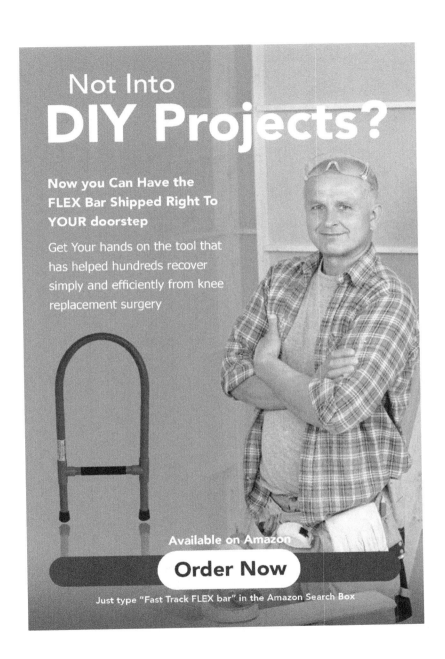

Made in the USA
Middletown, DE
26 September 2023

39477449R00046